ANGINA PECTORIS RELIEF

Effective Lifestyle Techniques to Alleviate Chest Discomfort and Improve Heart Function (Heart Health Handbook)

Isabella White

Copyright © 2024 by Isabella White.

Disclaimer: *The information in this book is based on the author's research, opinions, and experiences. It is not intended to replace professional medical advice or treatment. The reader should regularly consult a physician for any health issues and always seek the advice of a physician before modifying diet, supplement, or exercise regimens. The author and publisher shall have neither liability nor responsibility to any person or entity concerning any loss or damage related to the information contained in this book. The information provided is general and may not apply to every individual. Any reliance on the information contained herein is solely at the reader's risk.*

Table of Contents

Introduction

Chest pain and discomfort are common complaints that affect millions of people worldwide. While there are many potential causes, one of the most concerning is angina pectoris, a condition where reduced blood flow to the heart leads to chest tightness and pain. Though not a disease itself, angina is a symptom of underlying heart problems and a warning sign that you may be at increased risk of a heart attack or stroke.

If you or a loved one suffers from frequent angina episodes, you know how frightening and disruptive this pain can be. The uncomfortable pressure and squeezing sensations make carrying out normal daily activities difficult. You may limit physical exertion and social engagements to avoid triggering an attack. In severe cases, angina can progress without warning and become a chronic issue that significantly impacts quality of life.

The good news is that lifestyle changes and self-care techniques can go a long way toward banishing angina and promoting heart health. You have more power than you realize to reduce the frequency and severity of angina episodes and restore comfort and confidence. This book will be your guide to taking back control of your health.

Within these pages, we will explore the anatomical causes of angina and risk factors that may contribute to its development. You will learn what happens inside the body during an angina episode and why certain triggers can set off chest pain. Understanding physiology will help you identify your triggers and patterns.

Next, we will dive into many practical lifestyle measures focused on diet, exercise, sleep, stress management, and more. You will discover balanced, sustainable techniques to improve cardiovascular health from the inside out. These include nutritional strategies to support the heart, physical activity guidelines for your activity level, stress-busting practices to promote relaxation, and advice on optimizing sleep quality and consistency.

With the right lifestyle approach, most angina sufferers can substantially reduce the frequency and intensity of chest pain episodes. For many, bothersome angina fades into the background rather than dictating their choices.

No two patients are alike, so recommendations are tailored to their needs and abilities. You can assemble your customized "angina relief toolkit" based on your unique situation and areas you are ready to work on first. Small steps can lead to significant improvements.

While lifestyle techniques should be the foundation of any angina treatment plan, medication, and other medical therapies still play an important role in more severe cases. You will find a primer on current medical options and how they can complement self-care. Work closely with your physician for the most effective integrated approach.

Take heart, knowing that relief is within reach. With commitment to heart-healthy living and the practical advice in this book, you can break free from the limitations of angina and reclaim comfort, confidence, and quality of life. The road to lasting change starts here.

Chapter 1

Understanding Angina Pectoris

What is Angina Pectoris?

Angina pectoris refers to squeezing, pressure-like chest pain or discomfort when blood and oxygen flow to the heart muscle is temporarily reduced. It is not a disease in and of itself but rather a symptom of underlying heart problems that limit adequate oxygenation of the heart muscle.

Specifically, angina arises when the coronary arteries that supply the heart with its blood flow become narrowed or partially blocked. This typically occurs due to a buildup of fatty plaque deposits within the artery walls, known as atherosclerosis. Blood has trouble getting through as the passageways narrow, especially during increased cardiac demand.

When the heart is not receiving enough oxygen-rich blood to meet its needs at a given moment, you feel the chest discomfort, tightness, or pain termed angina pectoris, with "pec" referring to the chest and "angina" to the choking sensation. It may feel like uncomfortable pressure, squeezing, fullness, or pain in the center of the chest. Some also sense shoulder, arm, neck, jaw, or back pain. Angina attacks are usually fairly short-lived, lasting just 2 to 10 minutes in most cases.

There are a few forms angina can take:

- Stable angina is the most common, occurring in predictable patterns and with similar pain levels each time. It comes on with exertion or stress and goes away with rest. Walking, exercising, or getting overly emotional can trigger stable angina.
- Unstable angina is unexpected, occurs at rest, and is often more severe or prolonged. It is a warning sign of worsening coronary artery disease.
- Variant (Prinzmetal) angina occurs at rest with no obvious triggers, caused by coronary artery spasms rather than plaque. The pain pattern varies.

- Microvascular angina happens when the smaller coronary vessels constrict, with few or no large blockages. Women are more often affected.

Regardless of type, angina results from the heart's inability to get as much oxygen-rich blood as it needs to work properly. It should never be ignored, as it implies you have significantly reduced heart blood flow that could lead to a heart attack or irregular rhythms if unaddressed. That being said, stable angina with a predictable pattern is less concerning than sudden and intense chest pain.

Angina is sometimes confused with other causes of chest discomfort, like gastroesophageal reflux disease (GERD), muscle strains, pinched nerves, or anxiety. However, true angina tends to feel like a squeezing, pressing, or crushing sensation directly behind the breastbone. It may also radiate to the left shoulder and arm in many cases. GERD and muscle pain feel more like burning, sharp, or stabbing discomfort. Talk to your doctor if you are uncertain whether you experience true angina versus another cause of chest symptoms.

The key characteristics that differentiate angina pectoris from non-cardiac chest pain are its association with exertion or emotional stress, the short duration of episodes, and relief with rest. Making a note of these patterns is helpful when discussing with your physician whether your chest discomfort stems from heart disease versus other potential factors. An accurate diagnosis is the critical first step to getting appropriate treatment.

The Causes and Risk Factors

Angina pectoris does not arise independently but is a consequence of an underlying heart disease that limits oxygen supply to the cardiac muscle. The most common cause is atherosclerotic heart disease, where fatty deposits build up inside the arteries, feeding the heart and impeding blood flow. This process can begin early in life. Over time, the passageways narrow to the point where blood has trouble getting through, especially during surges in cardiac demand.

Atherosclerosis and progressive blocking of the coronary arteries explain why angina pectoris becomes more common with advancing age. By age 65, around 5% of women and 10% of men experience angina. Age itself is a risk factor, as are the following:

1. **Family history:** Genetic tendencies toward high cholesterol, hypertension, and heart disease increase angina risk.

2. **Smoking:** Chemicals in tobacco smoke injure artery walls. Nicotine also raises the heart rate and tightens blood vessels.

3. **High blood cholesterol:** Excess LDL cholesterol in the blood sticks to damaged arterial walls and builds up over time.

4. **Hypertension:** High blood pressure strains the heart and damages blood vessels. It often coincides with atherosclerosis.

5. **Diabetes:** Chronically high blood sugar corrodes arteries and the heart itself. Most diabetics have atherosclerosis.

6. **Overweight or obesity:** Excess body fat, especially around the abdomen, raises the risk of developing heart disease risk factors like high cholesterol, hypertension, and diabetes.

7. **Physical inactivity:** Lack of regular physical activity contributes to obesity, high blood pressure, diabetes, and atherosclerosis. Exercise is protective.

8. **Chronic stress:** Extended emotional stress boosts heart rate, constricts arteries, and aggravates other risk factors. Managing stress is beneficial.

9. **Nutritional factors:** Diets high in saturated fat, trans fat, salt, and processed carbohydrates while low in antioxidants promote atherosclerosis. A heart-healthy diet reduces risk substantially.

While atherosclerosis is by far the most frequent cause, angina can also arise from:

- Severe narrowing of the aortic valve at the outlet of the heart
- An aortic aneurysm puts pressure on the coronary arteries
- Coronary artery spasm and Prinz metal's variant angina
- Coronary artery dissection or tears
- Blood clots block the coronary arteries.
- Anemia or other blood disorders leading to lower oxygen-carrying capacity
- Cardiomyopathy that thickens or stiffens the heart muscle

The leading modifiable causes to focus on are atherosclerosis risk factors. Smoking cessation, blood pressure control, lowering elevated cholesterol, maintaining a healthy body weight, eating well, and exercising regularly all help prevent angina by promoting healthy arteries and heart function. Even if you already have developed angina, addressing risk factors helps stabilize or even reverse its course. Work with your physician on appropriate lifestyle improvements and medications as needed.

Symptoms of Angina Pectoris and How it is Diagnosed

The hallmark of angina pectoris is chest discomfort, described as squeezing, pressure, tightness, crushing, or pain. It often starts behind the breastbone but may radiate to the left shoulder, left arm, neck, back, or jaw. Some people sense pain only in these other areas. Discomfort from true angina usually lasts 2 to 10 minutes and goes away with rest.

Other signs and symptoms include:

- Shortness of breath along with chest discomfort
- Nausea, sweating, dizziness, or weakness are signs of reduced blood flow.
- A faster or irregular heartbeat during an angina episode

- Discomfort triggered by physical exertion, emotional stress, or exposure to cold and relieved by rest
- Worsening, prolonged pain that is not fully relieved by rest (unstable angina)

Angina tends to follow a pattern with each individual. Note details like your activity level when it strikes, location and type of pain, triggers, duration, and relieving factors. Stable angina comes on predictably with certain activities and resolves fully with rest. Unstable angina occurs unexpectedly and feels more severe.

Tell your doctor if you experience new, worsening, or changing chest discomfort patterns. Unexpected angina, especially at rest, suggests a worsening blockage that could lead to a heart attack and needs prompt medical attention. Call 911 immediately for chest pain that does not improve quickly with rest.

Physicians consider symptoms, medical history, risk factors, and test results to diagnose angina. Initial testing often includes:

- Physical exam—listening to the heart and lungs

- EKG to look for heart rhythm abnormalities and evidence of prior heart damage.
- Blood tests check cholesterol levels, blood cell counts, and markers of heart muscle injury.
- Exercise stress test monitoring—EKG changes and symptoms with exertion
- Echocardiogram using ultrasound to examine the heart's structure and function
- Coronary angiogram—visualizing the coronary arteries for blockages via injected dye
- CT coronary angiogram or coronary artery calcium scoring scan to reveal plaque in the arteries
- Cardiac MRI to assess heart structure, function, and scarring

These tests help clarify if your chest discomfort stems from insufficient heart blood flow rather than lung, muscle, or nerve issues. The pattern of discomfort is also telling—true angina comes on with exertion and goes away quickly with rest. Your doctor can determine whether your symptoms align with angina versus other potential causes. Accurate diagnosis is key to proper management.

Conventional Medical Treatments

While lifestyle improvement should serve as the foundation for managing angina pectoris, medication and procedures often play an important role. Anti-angina drugs, surgery to open blocked arteries, and occasionally implanted devices help control symptoms and improve heart blood flow.

Medications used include:

1. **Nitroglycerin:** Taken by mouth or under the tongue, it rapidly opens arteries to improve blood flow and relieve acute angina episodes.
2. **Beta-blockers:** Help reduce heart workload by slowing the heart rate and lessening the force of contraction. This reduces oxygen demand.
3. **Calcium channel blockers:** Relax coronary arteries to improve blood flow to the heart and relieve angina.
4. **Ranolazine:** Decreases angina attacks, likely by improving blood flow to areas with low oxygen.
5. **ACE inhibitors:** Lower blood pressure and may also open up blood vessels. It is helpful for stable angina.

6. **Statins:** Lower LDL "bad" cholesterol to help prevent further plaque buildup and improve outcomes.

Aspirin is also frequently prescribed to help prevent blood clot formation in areas of plaque. Your doctor will determine which, if any, medications are appropriate for your case based on efficacy and possible side effects. The goal is to find the most effective regimen with minimal side effects.

If lifestyle measures and medication do not adequately control angina, procedures to restore blood flow may be warranted. Common options include:

1. **Angioplasty with stent placement:** A catheter with a tiny balloon is threaded to the blocked artery and inflated to compress the plaque. A mesh tube, a stent, is usually inserted to open the artery.
2. **Coronary artery bypass grafting:** Blood flow is rerouted around severely blocked arteries using a healthy vein or artery from elsewhere in the body.
3. **Enhanced external counterpulsation (EECP):** Involves inflatable cuffs around the legs that inflate and deflate to move blood through the arteries in

time with the heartbeat. This can encourage the formation of new small blood vessels.

For cases, refractory to other treatments, occasional surgical procedures include trans myocardial laser revascularization and gene or stem cell therapy. As a last resort, implantable devices like pacemakers and internal cardioverter defibrillators may help manage arrhythmias and heart failure associated with severe angina.

Work closely with your cardiovascular team to determine the need for medications, surgical interventions, or device implantation to complement lifestyle modification. An integrated approach offers the best results. The latest procedures can provide dramatic relief, but most still require the diligent self-care covered in the following chapters to work optimally.

Outlook and Prognosis

The outlook for angina pectoris varies substantially based on underlying heart disease severity and treatment responsiveness. Mildly stable angina is well-controlled with lifestyle changes, and medication generally has a good prognosis. However, uncontrolled angina indicates compromised heart blood flow that could lead to a heart attack, arrhythmias, or heart failure if left unaddressed.

Many patients with mild angina experience few symptoms as long as they avoid triggers and take medications as prescribed. With attentive self-care and medical management, angina can remain stable for many years for some individuals. The prognosis is most favorable when atherosclerosis progression is halted or reversed through heart-healthy lifestyle habits.

However, without adequate treatment, chronic stable angina tends to worsen over the next 3–5 years. Unstable angina presents a more severe short-term risk. Frequent, unexpected episodes suggest a high-grade blockage that could fully occlude at any time, resulting in a heart attack. The first 2 months after unstable angina begins are the highest-risk period. Swift medical intervention is warranted.

Angina is also linked with higher mortality. The more frequent and severe the episodes, the poorer the outlook. However, optimal medical therapy and diligent lifestyle modification can significantly improve the prognosis. Key factors that affect the outlook include:

1. **Number of coronary arteries affected:** Single-vessel disease carries the most favorable outlook. The more arteries have blockages, the higher the risk.
2. **Severity of blockages:** Partial obstruction is better than critical narrowing. A complete occlusion requires urgent revascularization.
3. **The presence of collateral blood vessels**: Extra vessels supplying the heart muscle reduce ischemia.
4. **Left ventricular function:** Preserved pumping ability is ideal. Weakness portends heart failure.
5. **Other medical conditions:** Good control of diabetes, blood pressure, and other diseases improves the prognosis.
6. **Treatment adherence:** Consistent lifestyle improvement and medication use leads to better outcomes.
7. **Cessation of smoking:** This halts the progression of atherosclerosis.

With attentive self-care under a doctor's supervision, even patients with advanced angina can stabilize and improve their condition. However, without adequate treatment, the risk of heart attack, arrhythmias, and death rises significantly. Progression must be addressed.

If lifestyle changes are insufficient to control symptoms, procedures to open blocked arteries or implantable devices often become necessary. This reduces the supply-demand mismatch in oxygenation of the heart muscle that underlies angina.

Angina prognosis varies widely based on the severity of atherosclerosis, the presence of collateral circulation, treatment compliance, and the control of other diseases. Mildly stable angina generally carries a good outlook, but all angina must be adequately managed due to the risk of heart attack and reduced lifespan if unaddressed. Lifestyle improvement and medical treatment can make a major difference.

Chapter 2

Lifestyle Changes for Preventing Angina

Improving Diet and Nutrition

Diet and nutrition play a central role in preventing and managing angina pectoris. Controlling risk factors like high cholesterol, diabetes, excess weight, and hypertension through proper eating habits goes a long way toward promoting heart health and avoiding angina. Emphasize whole, minimally processed foods over convenience items whenever possible.

Focus first on limiting the intake of foods that directly damage arteries and worsen atherosclerosis. These include:

1. **Saturated and trans fats:** Found in fatty red meats, processed meats, fried items, baked goods, and some dairy products. Avoid it when possible.

2. **Added sugars:** High intake spikes blood sugar and insulin, promoting diabetes and arterial damage. Limit sweets, soda, juices, desserts, and the like.

3. **Refined grains:** Lack of fiber and worsening of blood sugar control. Opt for whole grains like oats, brown rice, quinoa, and 100% whole wheat bread.

4. **Excess salt:** Boosts blood pressure in salt-sensitive individuals. Avoid adding extra salt to the table.

5. **Processed convenience foods:** Packed with salt, sugar, low-quality fats, and preservatives while low in nutrients. Make home-cooked meals instead, when feasible. Moderation is key if you rely on frozen meals.

Instead, emphasize heart-healthy foods like:

1. **Fruits and vegetables:** Packed with antioxidants, fiber, minerals, and plant compounds that reduce inflammation and improve arterial function. Aim for 8–10 servings per day.

2. **Lean proteins:** Fish, skinless poultry, low-fat dairy products, legumes, nuts, and seeds. Build meals around these instead of red meat.

3. **Whole grains:** Choose 100% whole wheat, oats, brown rice, quinoa, and the like over refined versions. They are rich in B vitamins and fiber.

4. **Healthy fats:** Swap saturated fats for monounsaturated fats like olive and canola oils, avocados, nuts, and seeds. Oily fish provide anti-inflammatory omega-3 fats.

5. **Herbs, spices, and teas:** Contain antioxidant and anti-inflammatory compounds that boost heart health. Basil, garlic, ginger, turmeric, green tea, and hibiscus tea are great choices.

6. **Dark chocolate:** High in flavonoids with antioxidant effects. Stick to at least 70% cacao.

7. **Red wine:** Polyphenols may boost HDL cholesterol and reduce clotting when consumed in moderation. Limit to 1 glass per day with dinner if desired.

Work with a nutritionist or registered dietitian to craft a personalized heart-healthy diet that accounts for your caloric needs, medication use, and other medical conditions like diabetes or kidney disease. Small, sensible changes sustained over time have the greatest impact.

Increasing Physical Activity

Regular physical activity is a cornerstone of heart health and prevents angina. Exercise reduces atherosclerosis risk factors, relieves stress, and improves cardiovascular fitness. Aim for 150 minutes per week of moderate or 75 minutes of vigorous activity, plus muscle-strengthening exercises at least 2 days per week. Consult your doctor to ensure safety.

Aerobic exercise gets your heart pumping and controls blood pressure, blood sugar, weight, and cholesterol. Options include walking, jogging, cycling, swimming, rowing, aerobics classes, and more. Start slow and gradually increase duration and intensity. Warm up first and cool down afterward. Use a fitness tracker to monitor your heart rate and calories burned. Moderate exercise should raise your heart rate but still allow you to converse.

Strength training is also key; muscles will waste away without it, slowing metabolism. Weight lifting, resistance bands, bodyweight exercises like push-ups and crunches, yoga, and other muscle-building activities help maintain muscle mass. This becomes especially important as we get older. Two 30-minute strength sessions per week are a good goal.

Other helpful types of activity include:

1. **High-intensity interval training (HIIT):** Alternate short bursts of intense activity with lower-intensity recovery. Provides cardiovascular benefits efficiently.
2. **Tai chi:** This martial art improves stamina, strength, balance, and flexibility through flowing movements. It reduces stress as well.
3. **Yoga:** Builds strength, flexibility, and balance. focuses on breathing and meditation to lower stress hormones. Gentle types like Hatha yoga are good for beginners.
4. **Pilates:** Targets the core muscles using controlled movements and weights. It helps posture and joint health.
5. **Walking:** A simple way to start that requires no equipment. Work up to brisk 30-minute daily walks.

Any movement is better than remaining sedentary. Start slowly and focus on consistency rather than intensity at first. Over time, gradually challenge yourself to increase the duration, frequency, or intensity. Vary your workouts to prevent boredom. Enlist a friend, take classes, or use smartphone apps to stay motivated.

Always talk to your doctor before significantly increasing your activity level, especially if you already have angina or heart disease. Certain precautions, like avoiding extreme temperatures or taking nitroglycerin before exercising, may be advised. Build up slowly and learn to monitor your body's response. Report any concerning symptoms promptly. With guidance, most people can safely increase their fitness levels.

Physical activity is one of the most effective ways to prevent angina by reducing risk factors, controlling weight, and making the heart and blood vessels more resilient. Find activities you enjoy and make them a part of your daily routine.

Smoking Cessation

If you smoke or use tobacco products, quitting is one of the single most important steps you can take to avoid developing angina pectoris and improve your cardiovascular prognosis. Tobacco use is a major reversible risk factor for atherosclerosis and coronary artery disease, leading to angina. Quitting halts the progression of arterial damage and reduces heart attack risk quickly.

Cigarette smoking promotes angina and heart attacks in several ways:

- The nicotine in tobacco constricts blood vessels, reducing oxygen supply to the heart muscle. Carbon monoxide binds to hemoglobin, further limiting oxygen-carrying capacity.
- Chemicals in cigarette smoke injure the delicate endothelial cells lining the arteries, leading to atherosclerotic plaque buildup.
- Smoking raises blood pressure and heart rate, increasing the heart's workload.
- Tobacco impairs HDL "good" cholesterol while modifying LDL cholesterol to a more damaging form.
- Cigarettes induce inflammation and oxidative stress throughout the circulatory system.
- Smoking is linked to blood clots forming over areas of arterial plaque rupture that can wholly obstruct vessels.

The toxins in tobacco smoke exacerbate every step of atherosclerosis progression. This greatly heightens the risk of developing angina pectoris, heart attacks, strokes, and peripheral artery disease, leading to amputations or critical organ damage.

Fortunately, quitting smoking brings rapid benefits:

- Within 1 day, blood pressure and heart rate decrease.
- After 2–3 weeks, lung function and circulation start improving.
- In 1–9 months, coughing, shortness of breath, and heart disease risks are reduced.
- After 5 years, the heart attack risk drops to about half that of a smoker.
- After 10–15 years, the risk of stroke and heart disease returns to near that of someone who never smoked.

While long-term heavy smoking does cause some permanent arterial damage, quitting halts the rapid progression and brings the body remarkable healing over time. It is never too late to quit.

Combining counseling, nicotine replacement, prescription cessation medication, and support groups provides the greatest success. Ask your doctor about appropriate options to help you quit tobacco for good. The benefits for your heart health will be immense.

Managing Stress and Anxiety

Emotional stress and anxiety negatively impact the heart and vascular system if they are severe and sustained over time. Managing stress effectively reduces anginal chest pain and keeps arteries healthy. Make lifestyle adjustments to promote relaxation and inner calm.

When we feel pressured or threatened, the body activates the sympathetic nervous system, releasing stress hormones like adrenaline and cortisol. This accelerates the heart rate and constricts blood vessels, simultaneously increasing oxygen demand and reducing supply to the heart. Emotional distress can trigger angina episodes.

Stress and anxiety contribute to angina risk indirectly as well. Chronic stress promotes overeating, smoking, inactivity, disrupted sleep, and other unhealthy habits. It also increases systemic inflammation linked to atherosclerosis.

Try these strategies to improve stress management and resilience:

- Identify your personal stress triggers and patterns using a journal or app. Notice when you feel rising tension.

- Practice abdominal breathing—slow, regular, deep breaths from the diaphragm. This taps the parasympathetic relaxation response.

- Try meditation, visualization, body scans, or mantras to enter a calm, focused state and clear anxious thoughts. Start with just 5–10 minutes daily. Apps can help guide you.

- Do gentle yoga or tai chi to link breath, movement, and meditation.

- Spend time outdoors walking or hiking. Nature is calming.

- Listen to music, read an uplifting book, or enjoy an inspiring podcast.

- Talk to supportive friends and family who listen well without judgment.

- Consider counseling or a support group to learn coping techniques if stress feels overwhelming.

- Make time for beloved hobbies that absorb your attention fully.

- Prioritize adequate sleep and limit stimulants like caffeine.

- Eat a balanced diet with plenty of antioxidant-rich plant foods to reduce inflammation.

Stress is unavoidable, but you have power over your responses. With practice, you can learn to interrupt automatic anxious thoughts and consciously relax your body when overwhelmed. This reduces the toll that stress takes on your heart and overall health. Be patient and persistent in finding the right stress management approach for you.

Monitoring Weight and Body Composition

Excess body weight, especially abdominal and visceral fat, significantly increases the risk of developing angina pectoris. Carrying extra pounds strains the cardiovascular system and promotes insulin resistance, high cholesterol, hypertension, and systemic inflammation—all contributing factors to angina and atherosclerosis. Monitoring your weight and body composition aids in prevention.

While scales have their place, they do not distinguish between healthy lean mass and unhealthy body fat. Focus on maintaining a proper waist circumference and having a body composition with higher muscle than fat percentages.

These are stronger predictors of heart health than weight alone.

The ideal waist circumference is under 40 inches for men and under 35 inches for women when measuring just above the hips. Larger waist sizes correlate to dangerous visceral fat surrounding organs. This contributes more to insulin resistance, metabolic syndrome, and cardiovascular disease than subcutaneous fat beneath the skin.

There are a few options for periodically assessing body composition:

- Skinfold calipers measure fat layer thickness at different body sites. This approximates the total body fat percentage. A trainer can help with proper technique. Shoot for under 25% body fat for men and under 31% for women.

- Based on their different properties, bioelectrical impedance scales pass a mild current through your body to estimate fat versus lean tissue. These are affordable but less precise than other methods.

- Underwater weighing is considered the "gold standard" but requires specialized equipment. You are weighed repeatedly while submerged in a tank, and the water displacement is used to calculate lean tissue vs. fat tissue mass.

- DEXA scans pass two X-ray beams of different energy levels through the body to gauge fat, muscle, and bone density. This is very accurate but also expensive.

Monitoring body composition periodically helps maintain adequate muscle and avoid excess fat, especially in the abdominal region, which has the greatest health impacts. Speak to your physician about appropriate targets for your age, sex, and body type. Losing even 5–10% of your initial weight pays big dividends for your heart health.

Optimizing Sleeping Habits

Getting adequate, high-quality sleep consistently is vital for heart health and the prevention of angina pectoris. Adults should aim for 7-9 hours of sleep per night. Poor or insufficient sleep negatively impacts blood pressure, blood sugar control, inflammation, appetite regulation, and artery function—all risk factors for angina. Prioritize good sleep hygiene.

Try these tips to improve your sleep:

- Maintain a consistent sleep schedule, even on weekends. Wake up and go to bed at the same times daily. This stabilizes the circadian rhythm that governs sleep.

- Develop relaxing pre-bedtime rituals like reading, gentle yoga, or bathing. This tells your body that it is time for sleep.

- Make sure your bedroom is comfortable, relaxed, quiet, and dark. Upgrade your mattress if needed.

- Avoid electronic devices and bright lights before bed; these suppress melatonin production.

- Limit caffeine, alcohol, and heavy meals too close to bedtime. Caffeine and alcohol disrupt sleep quality.

- Reduce fluid intake 2 hours before bed to decrease nighttime trips to the bathroom.

- Try magnesium, melatonin, or chamomile tea supplements if needed, but start with the lowest effective dose.

- Stick to your sleep schedule as much as possible during illnesses or times of stress. Maintaining rhythm helps.

- Rule out any underlying sleep disorders, like sleep apnea, by talking with your doctor. These must be addressed.
- Get exposure to natural bright light first thing in the morning and during the daytime to regulate rhythm.

Pay attention to how you feel after different amounts of sleep. Most adults need at least 7 hours to function optimally. Prioritize sleep over late-night television or social media. Allow extra time to wind down before bed.

Consistent sleep deficiency stresses the body, impairs focus and judgment, and increases angina risk. Do not dismiss the importance of quality sleep for maintaining heart health. Discuss any persistent troubles with your doctor and be evaluated for sleep apnea or other disorders if necessary. Adjusting your lifestyle and environment for better sleep has tremendous benefits for your health and well-being.

Chapter 3

Alternative Therapies and Complementary Approaches

Mind-Body Practices like Yoga & Meditation

Mind-body modalities that cultivate relaxation while connecting the breath, body, and mind show promise as complementary therapies for managing angina pectoris. Yoga, meditation, tai chi, qigong, and guided imagery are all practices that help to counteract the "fight or flight" stress response that strains the heart. Performing them consistently helps relieve anxiety and chest discomfort while promoting overall well-being.

Yoga encompasses physical postures and poses combined with deep breathing and meditation. It builds strength, flexibility, and balance while quieting the mind. Iyengar and Hatha yoga are gentle styles well-suited for beginners. Yoga helps:

- Improve oxygenation efficiency, allowing the cardiovascular system to function better under stress.
- Increase chest wall expansion and lung capacity through breathing exercises. This also boosts the oxygen supply to the heart muscle.
- Lower blood pressure, resting heart rate, and cholesterol levels.
- Enhance parasympathetic nervous system activity to reduce stress hormones like cortisol.
- Reduce inflammation and improve coronary blood vessel function.

Simple meditation practices involve sitting quietly while focusing on the breath, an image, or a repeated word or phrase (mantra). This elicits deep relaxation and counters anxiety. Meditation has been shown to:

- Reduce blood pressure, heart rate, chest pain episodes, and the need for angina medication.
- Lessens stress hormone levels and dampens nervous system arousal.
- Potentially give rise to new tiny collateral coronary blood vessels that "bypass" blockages.

- Help patients disengage from pain sensations during angina episodes.

Mind-body modalities should serve as an adjunct to, not a replacement for, medical therapies and lifestyle changes. Work with a qualified instructor and get your doctor's approval before starting. Begin gently and gradually increase the duration. Be consistent for maximum benefits. Yoga, meditation, and similar practices benefit cardiovascular health while providing psychological benefits to cope with angina as well.

Herbal Remedies and Supplements

Certain herbal remedies and nutritional supplements show modest benefits for managing angina pectoris when used appropriately in conjunction with lifestyle changes and medical treatment. The available scientific evidence for most is limited. Do not use herbs or supplements as a substitute for medications prescribed by your doctor.

Some examples include:

1. **Ginkgo biloba:** This extract from the ancient Chinese ginkgo tree may modestly enhance blood flow and oxygenation in ischemic areas based on its antioxidant and anti-inflammatory effects. Studies

show mixed results. It generally does not reduce angina attacks but may slightly improve exercise time until cramping pain occurs. Take only under medical supervision.

2. **Hawthorn berry:** Hawthorn contains flavonoids that help dilate blood vessels, improve circulation, and reduce plaque formation. Some studies suggest a mild benefit for chronic stable angina, but the effects are inconsistent. It may interact with heart medications.

3. **Coenzyme Q10:** Found naturally in the body, coQ10 plays a role in cell energy production. Some research indicates that coQ10 supplementation could benefit certain patients with angina, heart failure, and other cardiovascular diseases. Discuss with your doctor.

4. **Magnesium:** Angina and certain blood pressure medications may deplete magnesium. Supplements may help correct low levels, which could increase blood flow and oxygenation. More evidence is needed.

5. **L-carnitine:** This amino acid is involved in energy metabolism. L-carnitine supplements could improve exercise tolerance slightly in chronic stable angina,

but they do not decrease angina attacks—there is little harm in trying under medical guidance.

6. **Omega-3 fatty acids:** In fish oil, omega-3s modestly lower triglycerides, improve endothelial function, and reduce inflammation. These effects may benefit some angina patients. Use high-quality supplements only.

7. **Garlic:** Long used in folk medicine, garlic mildly reduces blood pressure, cholesterol, and platelet aggregation. This could benefit angina treatment. Eating fresh garlic as food is likely more effective than supplements alone.

Herbs and supplements should never serve as an alternative to prescribed medications and lifestyle changes. Effects tend to be modest at best. Tell your doctor about any complementary approaches you wish to try to ensure they are appropriate for your situation and will not interact with other treatments. More rigorous research is still needed.

Acupuncture and Acupressure

Acupuncture and acupressure, key components of Traditional Chinese Medicine, may offer modest benefits as complementary techniques for preventing and managing chronic stable angina. They are not appropriate for unstable angina requiring urgent care. Always work with a licensed practitioner.

Acupuncture involves inserting very thin needles into specific points on the body to manipulate the energy flow, or "qi." Traditional theory holds that blocked qi causes pain and organ dysfunction. Acupuncture aims to open qi flow to restore health to affected areas. Systematic reviews conclude:

- Acupuncture is moderately effective in improving angina symptoms and quality of life.
- It may modestly lower the frequency of angina attacks and the use of anti-angina medication versus no acupuncture.
- The benefits seem greatest for those with an initial angina severity of moderate or higher.
- The impact on reducing mortality risk or the need for invasive procedures is inconclusive.

Typical acupuncture protocols involve needle insertion at 4–8 points on the wrists, legs, neck, and chest areas to improve heart qi. Sessions last 20–30 minutes and are usually repeated weekly or biweekly. Mild soreness, bleeding, or bruising sometimes occur. The risk of serious side effects is low when performed by licensed acupuncturists.

Acupressure applies targeted finger pressure instead of needles to stimulate the same acupuncture points and meridians. This therapy is safe and easily self-administered, providing a non-invasive alternative. Users report decreased chest discomfort. It may be helpful as adjunctive symptom relief.

For chronic stable angina patients willing to try, acupuncture and acupressure are reasonably safe options that could improve quality of life and supplement conventional treatments. However, reductions in angina frequency and severity are generally modest. Get your cardiologist's opinion before starting. More research is still needed.

Therapeutic Massage and Bodywork

Various therapeutic massage and bodywork forms offer potential benefits for angina pectoris patients, including reduced anxiety, lowered blood pressure, and improved heart rate variability. Always consult your cardiologist before starting massage therapy. Avoid it during unstable angina episodes.

The potential benefits of professional massage for heart health include the following:

- Decreased cortisol and norepinephrine are stress hormones that constrict blood vessels. Massage boosts mood-boosting serotonin and dopamine.
- Increased parasympathetic "rest and digest" nervous system activity reduces blood pressure and heart rate.
- Enhanced heart rate variability shows healthy autonomic function and the ability to handle stress.
- Improved coronary artery blood flow, especially in people with initially low flow rates.
- Reduced procedural anxiety, tension, and pain during angioplasty surgery—massage before surgery appears helpful.
- Lowered perceptions of angina pain when performed during episodes, likely by dampening pain signaling pathways.
- Decreased inflammatory signaling molecules are linked to atherosclerosis progression.

While study sample sizes are often limited, the consistency of observed benefits is encouraging. Massage techniques studied include Swedish massage, craniosacral therapy, reflexology, and massage directed at acupressure points. Benefits appear most pronounced with the first several weekly sessions.

Always obtain medical clearance before starting massage therapy, especially if you have unstable angina or other uncontrolled heart disease. Alert your massage therapist to any recent episodes or changes in your condition. Avoid compressing the chest directly over the sternum. Gentle touch and strokes improve comfort without affecting heart rate or circulation.

When incorporated wisely, massage and bodywork provide a helpful adjunct to standard angina care for many patients. Effects on circulation and stress reduction can enhance well-being and aid self-regulating heart health. Therapeutic massage serves as a safe, drug-free option to discuss with your cardiologist.

Chapter 4

Medications and Medical Procedures

Nitrates, Beta Blockers, Calcium Channel Blockers

In addition to lifestyle modifications, several medication classes effectively prevent angina attacks and improve blood flow to the heart. These include nitrates, beta-blockers, and calcium channel blockers. They are often prescribed in combination.

Nitrates (nitroglycerin):
- Work rapidly to dilate and relax blood vessels, increasing blood flow to the heart and quickly relieving acute angina episodes.
- They are available as short-acting pills, sprays, patches, and pastes for on-demand angina relief. Long-acting oral and patch formulations help prevent attacks.

- It helps reduce angina symptoms and improve exercise capacity when used regularly.
- It can cause side effects like headaches, dizziness, and low blood pressure. Tolerance to the effects may develop over time.

Beta-blockers:

- Block the effects of adrenaline to reduce heart rate, blood pressure, and workload on the heart. This decreases oxygen demand.
- They help with angina caused by physical exertion, emotional stress, or cold temperatures.
- Have been shown to reduce the frequency of angina episodes and improve exercise capacity.
- It can cause fatigue, sleep disturbances, and reduced exercise tolerance in some patients.

Calcium channel blockers:

- Prevent calcium from entering the heart and blood vessel cells, which relaxes arteries to enhance blood flow.
- It is a good option for patients who cannot tolerate beta-blockers well.
- Also, reduce the forcefulness of heart muscle contractions.

- It helps control blood pressure in addition to reducing angina episodes.
- It may cause constipation or ankle swelling in some patients.

Medications for angina often work best when used together. For example, combining a fast-acting nitrate for acute attacks with a beta blocker or calcium channel blocker for long-term prevention is more effective than a single drug. Work with your cardiologist to tailor the optimal medication regimen for your specific needs.

Angioplasty and Stent Placement

If lifestyle changes and medications are not enough to control angina symptoms, procedures to physically widen narrowed arteries often become necessary. Angioplasty with stent placement is the most frequently performed minimally invasive technique.

During angioplasty:

- A thin, flexible tube called a catheter is inserted through an artery (often in the groin or wrist) and carefully threaded to the site of the blockage.

- A tiny balloon at the tip is inflated, compressing the plaque against the artery wall to expand the passageway.

- A small metal mesh tube called a stent often remains in the newly opened area to help keep it patent. The stent expands like scaffolding when released.

- The procedure lasts 30–90 minutes. Patients are awake but sedated. Recovery typically involves 6–12 hours of monitoring.

- Around 90% of patients experience immediate relief of angina and chest pain once a procedure is successfully performed.

- Over several months, arteries sometimes narrow again due to additional plaque buildup. Repeat procedures may be needed.

Risks include bleeding, blood clots, heart attack, stroke, and infection. However, complications are relatively rare when performed by an experienced cardiologist. Medications like aspirin and blood thinners help reduce the risk of clotting.

Newer-generation drug-eluting stents release compounds to help minimize the regrowth and narrowing of scar tissue.

Studies show these provide long-term outcomes comparable to bypass in appropriate patients.

Angioplasty with stenting offers a minimally invasive option to quickly improve blood flow and symptoms when medication no longer adequately controls angina. It does not cure the underlying atherosclerosis. Aggressive lifestyle changes and medical management are still needed after the procedure. Discuss the risks and benefits with your interventional cardiologist.

Coronary Artery Bypass Grafting Surgery

Coronary artery bypass grafting (CABG) is an open-heart surgery that reroutes blood flow around severely blocked arteries to restore oxygen supply to the heart muscle. It is an option mainly for patients with left main coronary artery disease or complex multi-vessel blockages unresponsive to other treatments.

During CABG:

- The patient is put under general anesthesia, and the heart is temporarily stopped during the procedure.
- Blood flow is maintained through a heart-lung machine.

- Sections of a healthy artery or vein, often from the legs, are grafted from the aorta onto points past obstructions in the coronary arteries. This bypasses the blockages.

- Multiple grafts are usually required based on the number of affected arteries and the degree of blockage.

- Hospital stays average one week. A full recovery takes at least 12 weeks.

CABG benefits:

- Significantly reduces or eliminates angina and chest pain by improving blood flow to the heart muscle.

- Studies show that CABG slightly outperforms angioplasty at reducing mortality in certain patients, like those with diabetes and advanced coronary artery disease.

- Bypass grafts can maintain excellent blood flow in many patients for 10–15 years. Younger patients may require repeat procedures eventually as grafts age.

Complications include bleeding, infection, stroke, and adverse reactions to anesthesia. Proper patient selection and surgical expertise reduce risks. Regular exercise and aggressive risk factor modification after surgery are vital.

For symptomatic patients with coronary anatomy not amenable to angioplasty, CABG remains the definitive revascularization technique. Discuss options thoroughly with your cardiologist and cardiac surgeon. Combining needed bypass procedures with internal mammary artery grafts provides excellent long-term results.

Chapter 5

Tracking Symptoms and Finding Support

Keeping an Angina Diary to Track Symptoms and Monitor Progress

Keeping an ongoing log of your angina episodes and symptom patterns is one of the best ways to monitor your condition and determine how well treatment works. An angina diary helps you track attack frequency, severity, triggers, and relieving factors over time. Share it regularly with your doctor. Be sure to record:

- Date and time the angina episode started and stopped.
- Where you were and what you were doing when it began
- What physical or emotional trigger may have set it off?

- How severe would you rate the pain on a scale of 1–10?
- The exact location of the discomfort or pain
- How long did the attack last?
- What medications or rest helped relieve it?
- Any other associated symptoms like shortness of breath, sweating, or dizziness
- Notes on your stress level, recent activity, or diet surrounding the event.

Tracking details helps identify your triggers and patterns. For example, you may notice certain activities, times of day, or emotions tend to provoke angina, while rest or nitroglycerin tablets provide rapid relief. Communicating these details to your doctor allows for better customization of your treatment plan.

Rate attack severity using a simple 1 to 10 scale, with 10 being the most intense pain imaginable. Note if attacks increase in frequency or become more severe over time. Worsening patterns may necessitate medication adjustments or procedures to open clogged arteries.

An angina diary allows you to assess the impact of lifestyle changes and new medications on attack frequency and intensity. Improvement will be encouraging! Share your records with your doctor to collaboratively adjust therapy until your angina is well controlled.

With a daily notation habit, an angina diary provides an invaluable record of your progress in fighting this condition. It puts control in your hands.

Joining Patient Support Groups for Those Living with Angina Pectoris

In addition to the support of your medical team, connecting with other patients dealing with angina can help you feel less alone and more empowered to manage your condition. Support groups provide a forum to share experiences, helpful solutions, and encouragement in a judgment-free space. Reasons to consider joining an angina support group:

- Gain emotional support and motivation from others facing the same challenges. Realize you are not alone.
- Hear how other patients successfully limit and relieve their chest pain episodes with lifestyle tweaks and stress management.

- Learn about helpful resources like exercise regimens, counseling referrals, or home healthcare services tailored for angina patients.
- Feel comfortable discussing sensitive topics like anxiety over intimacy and physical activity after a diagnosis.
- Get informed about the latest research and technologies for detecting and treating heart disease from fellow patients' experiences.
- Find accountability partners to exchange healthy recipes, workout tips, and progress check-ins.

Support groups are available locally through hospital programs, health clinics, and national organizations like the American Heart Association and Angina.com. Search online databases to find in-person or virtual groups that fit your needs and schedule.

The camaraderie and wealth of shared knowledge provide a valuable supplement to your medical care. Support groups can help you stick to prescribed lifestyle changes and feel empowered rather than overwhelmed in your health journey.

However, always defer to your own doctor's advice over anecdotes. Follow their guidelines for allowable activities, diet, medications, and procedures. Take notes on group discussions to review with your cardiologist later.

With an attitude of learning and giving back, support groups help transform the angina journey from isolating to uplifting. You gain new friends who understand the challenges involved.

Communicating with Your Healthcare Team

Open, honest communication with your cardiologist, primary care doctor, nurses, and other healthcare team members is critically important for properly managing angina pectoris. Speak up with any concerns, and make sure you understand all aspects of your treatment plan.

Helpful tips for communicating with your providers:

- Come prepared to appointments with a list of questions and topics to discuss, including any new or worsening symptoms. Bring a notebook to record instructions.
- Share your angina diary detailing attack frequency, severity, triggers, relief measures, and how symptoms impact your daily life. Give updates on lifestyle modifications.

- Ask your doctor to explain test results, proposed treatments, medications and side effects, activity recommendations, and goals at your current management stage.

- Voice any fears or anxieties you have about your prognosis, treatment options, medication adherence, or day-to-day self-care so they can be addressed.

- Request extra time during office visits if needed. Let the office know beforehand if a translator service is required. Bring a trusted companion along if desired.

- Provide input on treatment decisions rather than passively agreeing. Make sure you understand the risks and benefits before consenting to procedures. Please share your preferences.

- Review what signs or symptoms require prompt medical attention, such as increased attack frequency or pain at rest. Know how best to reach your care team with urgent concerns.

- Ask who handles medication refill requests, pre-authorizations, appointment scheduling, and other administrative tasks so you can contact the appropriate person.

- Seek clarification if you are uncertain about any instructions before leaving appointments. Repeat important points to ensure understanding.
- Express appreciation to nurses, medical assistants, and other staff for the care they provide at each visit.

Speaking openly lets your cardiologist make fully informed recommendations tailored to your needs and preferences, improving adherence. You are an equal partner in care decisions. Do not hesitate to utilize your care team's knowledge and experience to achieve the best possible outcome.

Conclusion

If you or someone you love suffers from angina pectoris, take heart, knowing there are many effective strategies available to minimize chest pain and live fully. With lifestyle changes, medical treatment, symptom tracking, and support, most patients achieve excellent control of stable angina and positive health outcomes.

Ignoring or downplaying symptoms is risky, while assertive management grants comfort and confidence. Arm yourself with knowledge of angina's underlying causes and multi-pronged therapies proven to limit ischemic episodes and their intensity. Even complex multi-vessel diseases need not prevent enjoying life when properly addressed.

Implement heart-healthy nutrition, regular activity at your own pace, stress management practices, restorative sleep, and smoking cessation. Medications and procedures further optimize oxygen supply to overtaxed cardiac muscle. Keeping an angina diary helps customize treatment to your unique patterns. Support groups provide community and fresh ideas from fellow patients.

Partner closely with your cardiologist, nurses, therapists, and other providers. Speak up with questions and concerns. Follow prescribed regimens diligently while voicing your needs for any adjustments to improve symptom control or reduce medication side effects. Ongoing communication, self-care, and expert guidance offer the best chance of stability.

Take things day by day. Not every day will be pain-free, but with time, angina often transitions from a daily concern to just an occasional nuisance. There are still activities to enjoy and goals to work towards. Let angina motivate the development of healthier long-term habits rather than allow it to dictate restrictions. A fulfilling, active life remains possible.

Stay positive and be patient with the process. Small, consistent improvements build over weeks and months to increase stamina and well-being. With the right balance of self-care, medical treatment, and lifestyle adjustment, you can manage angina pectoris and feel like your energized self again. Keep the faith!

Glossary of Key Terms

Angina pectoris: Chest pain or discomfort that occurs when the heart muscle receives insufficient oxygenated blood flow. Often described as tightness, pressure, squeezing, or crushing pain.

Atherosclerosis: Buildup of fatty plaque deposits called atherosclerotic lesions within the artery walls. This narrows the vessels, restricting blood flow.

Arrhythmia: Abnormal heart rhythm. Angina increases the risk of arrhythmias, like atrial fibrillation.

Angioplasty: Procedure to widen narrowed arteries using a small balloon catheter pushed through the blood vessels to the blockage.

Beta-blockers: Medications that reduce the workload on the heart by slowing the heart rate and contraction force. Help prevent angina attacks.

Calcium channel blockers: Medications that relax and open coronary arteries by preventing calcium influx into cells.

Cardiomyopathy: Disease of the heart muscle that causes it to thicken, enlarge, or stiffen. This can restrict blood flow and cause angina.

Collateral circulation: Extra smaller blood vessels that can supply the heart muscle if major coronary arteries are very blocked. It helps reduce angina severity.

Coronary arteries: Arteries on the surface of the heart that supply oxygen-rich blood to the heart muscle. Blockages here cause angina.

CABG (Coronary Artery Bypass Grafting): Open-heart surgery uses vein or artery grafts to bypass severely blocked coronary arteries.

Endothelium: Inner cell layer lining the interior surface of blood vessels, subject to damage from high cholesterol, smoking, hypertension, etc.

Myocardial ischemia: Reduced blood flow to the heart muscle, leading to oxygen deprivation. Causes angina pain.

Nitrates: Fast-acting medications like nitroglycerin that rapidly dilate coronary arteries, relieving acute angina episodes.

Plaque: Accumulations of fat, cholesterol, calcium, and inflammatory cells that build up in artery walls. Plaque narrows the inside passageways.

Stenosis: Abnormal narrowing of a blood vessel. Coronary artery stenosis causes impaired blood flow that can precipitate angina.

Stent: A tiny metal mesh tube inserted into an artery during angioplasty to help keep the vessel stretched open and maintain blood flow.